I0703432

ANTI-AGING TREATMENT FOR BEGINNERS

Effective Skincare Routines, Natural Remedies, And Expert Tips For Youthful Skin

DR SAWYER DIEGO

Copyright © [2024] by [Dr. .Sawyer Diego]. All rights reserved.

Except for brief quotations included in critical reviews and certain other noncommercial uses allowed by copyright law, no part of this publication may be reproduced, distributed, or transmitted in any form or by any means, including photocopying, recording, or other electronic or mechanical methods, without the publisher's prior written permission.

DISCLAMER

Nothing in this book should be interpreted as medical advice; it is meant exclusively for educational reasons. Regarding their specific health issues and treatment options, readers are urged to speak with licensed healthcare professionals. The publisher and author disclaim all liability for any errors or omissions in the material provided, as well as for any negative effects that may arise from using or abusing the information. Although every attempt has been taken to guarantee that the material in this book is correct as of the date of publishing, new research may have superseded some of the content because medical knowledge is always changing. It is recommended that readers confirm the most recent medical recommendations and guidelines. The reader of this book undertakes to release the author and publisher from any claims or liabilities resulting from the use of this information, and understands and accepts the inherent risks connected with healthcare decisions.

TABLE OF CONTENTS

ABOUT THE BOOK

Understanding the biological inevitability of aging and how it affects each person differently due to genetic predispositions and environmental influences makes "Anti-Aging Treatment for Beginners" an invaluable resource for anyone looking to understand and effectively combat the natural processes of aging. This book demystifies aging by examining its underlying biological processes, including the roles of free radicals, antioxidants, genetics, hormones, and other important factors. By exploring these scientific foundations, readers gain a comprehensive understanding of why aging occurs and how it manifests uniquely in each individual.

The focus of this book is on the fundamental skincare routines and lifestyle changes that underpin anti-aging practices. It addresses common misconceptions about anti-aging treatments, dispelling myths to provide readers with accurate information. From creating a customized daily skincare routine to choosing products based on skin type, the book offers helpful guidance on cleansing, exfoliating, moisturizing, and the critical importance of sun protection.

A good chunk of the book is devoted to teaching readers about key anti-aging ingredients like retinoids, vitamin C, hyaluronic acid, and peptides. These ingredients are critical in revitalizing skin health and effectively battling signs of aging. Additionally, the guide emphasizes the importance of healthy lifestyle choices like proper diet, adequate hydration, regular exercise, and enough sleep, all of which help preserve youthful skin and general well-being.

In addition to skincare regimens and lifestyle modifications, the book offers a thorough overview of non-surgical and surgical anti-aging treatments. It covers a wide range of options available to address specific aging concerns, from chemical peels and microdermabrasion to laser therapies and facial massages. For those who are considering more advanced interventions, detailed information about surgical procedures like facelifts, botox, fillers, eyelid surgery, and liposuction is provided, along with considerations for men who face particular challenges in anti-aging care.

To maximize treatment efficacy, the book also highlights strategies for maintaining pH balance and choosing appropriate products based on skin type. It also provides expert advice and practical solutions to address common concerns like wrinkles, age spots, sagging skin, under-eye bags, and dark circles. Additionally, the guide offers tailored advice for different skin types, recognizing the diverse needs of dry, oily, sensitive, and combination skin.

The book highlights the global perspective on anti-aging research and provides insights into the innovations driving advancements in skincare and wellness worldwide. It looks towards the future, exploring emerging trends in anti-aging technology and treatments and highlighting the significance of customized skincare regimens and sustainable practices in the industry.

Whether you're just starting on your anti-aging journey or looking to improve your current regimen, "Anti-Aging Treatment for Beginners" is more than just a guide; it's an all-encompassing resource created to give readers the knowledge and tools needed to navigate the complexities of aging gracefully and confidently. It provides you with expert advice and actionable insights to help you achieve long-lasting skin health and vitality.

CHAPTER ONE

ANTI-AGING TREATMENT OVERVIEW

WHAT DOES AGING INCLUDE AND WHY DOES IT OCCUR?

Natural biological aging is defined by the slow deterioration of body processes and the appearance of visible changes in the skin, muscles, and organs. It is brought on by a confluence of genetic factors, environmental factors, and lifestyle decisions over time. The skin, in particular, experiences changes like decreased production of collagen and elastin, which causes wrinkles, sagging, and dryness. Internally, organs become less efficient, which affects general health and vitality.

Knowing the biological mechanisms of aging allows people to make educated decisions about skincare practices, diet, exercise, and medical interventions that slow down the effects of aging. This knowledge also empowers people to adopt customized preventive strategies and treatments that improve their quality of life as they age. Understanding aging helps people accept the inevitable nature of these changes while emphasizing proactive measures to maintain health and appearance.

THE SIGNIFICANCE OF ANTI-AGING THERAPIES

Anti-aging treatments are essential for maintaining a youthful appearance and improving overall health as one age. They take many different forms, ranging from skincare products and lifestyle modifications to cutting-edge medical procedures. The goals of these treatments are to minimize visible signs of aging, such as wrinkles and age spots, as well as to increase collagen production, improve skin elasticity, and stimulate cellular rejuvenation.

A proactive approach to anti-aging can not only improve physical appearance but also boost self-confidence and promote a healthy lifestyle that supports overall vitality. Early investment in anti-aging treatments can significantly delay the onset of visible aging and maintain skin health over the long term. Individuals can optimize their anti-aging efforts by integrating effective skincare routines, nutrition, exercise, and stress management techniques.

BASICS OF CHANGING ONE'S LIFESTYLE AND SKINCARE

A strong foundation of skincare and lifestyle practices that promote skin health and vitality is necessary for effective anti-aging. Daily routines like cleansing, moisturizing, and wearing sunscreen protect against UV damage, which is the main cause of premature aging. Eating a well-balanced diet high in vitamins, antioxidants, and essential fatty acids promotes cellular renewal and repair while fending off oxidative stress and inflammation that causes aging to accelerate.

Maintaining overall well-being and minimizing the effects of aging requires a shift in lifestyle, which includes regular exercise, getting enough sleep, and practicing stress management techniques like yoga or meditation. These habits not only improve skin health but also mental clarity, emotional balance, and sustained energy levels. By putting these foundational elements first, people can set the stage for long-lasting anti-aging treatments.

HOW THIS BOOK WILL DIRECT YOU

Through structured chapters, readers will learn step-by-step methods to develop customized anti-aging routines that suit their individual needs and preferences. This book is a comprehensive resource for beginners looking to navigate the complexities of anti-aging treatments with confidence and clarity. It offers practical insights into understanding the aging process, dispelling common myths, and outlining effective strategies for skincare and lifestyle adjustments.

This book provides comprehensive guidance on choosing skin care products, implementing dietary changes, incorporating exercise routines, and considering advanced treatments.

Whether you're new to anti-aging practices or looking to improve your current regimen, it gives you the knowledge and tools you need to achieve visible results and long-term skin health. By dissecting complex concepts into easily understood information, it empowers readers to make informed decisions about their anti-aging journey.

MYTHS PREVALENT IN ANTI-AGING

Myths regarding anti-aging treatments can cause uncertainty and inflated expectations. Examples of common misconceptions are that high-end products are inherently better, that skincare can reverse the effects of aging completely, and that genetics is the only factor that determines aging. In actuality, effective anti-aging necessitates a comprehensive approach that includes lifestyle changes, skincare, and occasionally customized professional interventions.

By busting myths, people can more easily separate fact from fiction and make well-informed decisions regarding their anti-aging journey. Knowing that long-lasting results stem from individualized care and consistent habits gives people the power to prioritize what works for their skin type and lifestyle, which in turn sets reasonable expectations and promotes a proactive attitude toward aging gracefully and healthily.

CHAPTER TWO
THE SCIENCE OF GETTING OLDER
AGING PROCESSES IN BIOLOGY

The biological changes that occur in our bodies as we age are responsible for a number of the biological changes that contribute to the aging process. One important factor is cellular aging, which is the process by which cells eventually lose their capacity to divide and function at their best. Over time, oxidative stress, inflammation, and the accumulation of DNA damage all play a role in this process. Another important factor is cellular senescence, which is the state in which cells stop dividing but continue to be metabolically active. Cells in this state can accumulate in tissues and contribute to age-related degenerative diseases.

Declining organ function is another important biological process: as we age, our heart, kidneys, and brain all experience structural and functional changes that result in reduced efficiency and increased susceptibility to disease. For instance, the heart muscles can stiffen and thicken, making it harder for them to pump blood efficiently; the brain also gradually loses connections between its neurons, which causes a gradual decline in memory and cognitive function.

The biological processes of aging also include hormonal changes. The endocrine system, which controls hormones, changes as we age, impacting metabolism, sexual function, and general health. For example, hormone levels such as testosterone, estrogen, and growth hormone decrease with age, affecting bone density, muscle mass, and reproductive health. Knowledge of these biological processes aids in understanding the complex processes of aging and directs the development of anti-aging strategies.

ELEMENTS THAT AFFECT AGING

The process of aging is impacted by a complex interplay of internal and external factors.

Genetic predispositions play a major role internally, as genetic variations can affect an individual's rate of aging and susceptibility to age-related diseases. Lifestyle choices, on the other hand, have a significant impact on aging. Stress management, exercise, sleep patterns, and diet all have an impact on how gracefully an individual ages.

In addition to socioeconomic factors, access to healthcare, and psychological well-being, aging outcomes also include environmental factors like pollution exposure, UV radiation, and lifestyle habits like smoking and excessive alcohol consumption. These factors accelerate aging processes by contributing to oxidative stress, inflammation, and DNA damage, which in turn accelerates cellular aging and increases the risk of chronic diseases.

By addressing modifiable risk factors and adopting healthy behaviors, individuals can mitigate the effects of aging and improve their quality of life as they age. By understanding these diverse influences on aging, people are better equipped to make choices that may slow down the aging process and enhance overall health and longevity.

RECOGNIZING ANTIOXIDANTS AND FREE RADICALS

This damage, known as oxidative stress, is a major factor in aging and age-related diseases like cancer, heart disease, and neurodegenerative disorders. Free radicals are unstable molecules that are produced during normal cellular metabolism and in response to environmental stressors like pollution and UV radiation. These molecules have unpaired electrons, which makes them highly reactive and capable of damaging cellular structures like proteins, lipids, and DNA.

To counteract the damaging effects of free radicals, antioxidants neutralize free radicals by donating electrons without becoming unstable themselves. Antioxidants can be found naturally in a variety of foods and dietary supplements. Examples of common antioxidants are vitamins C and E, beta-carotene, and selenium. By increasing their intake of antioxidants through diet and supplements, people can potentially slow down the aging process and improve their defenses against oxidative stress.

Maintaining cellular health and longevity requires a balance between the production of free radicals and antioxidants; oxidative damage can be mitigated and healthy aging can be promoted by a diet high in antioxidants and lifestyle choices that limit exposure to environmental pollutants.

GENETICS'S PART IN AGING

Genetic variations inherited from parent's impact the rate of cellular aging, an individual's susceptibility to age-related diseases, and their overall longevity. Certain genes are linked to higher risks of age-related diseases like Alzheimer's, cardiovascular disease, and some types of cancer, highlighting the genetic basis of aging outcomes. Genetics plays a fundamental role in how individuals age.

Environmental factors such as diet, exercise, stress, and exposure to toxins can modify gene expression patterns, impacting aging processes. For example, lifestyle choices that promote healthy gene expression patterns may delay the onset of age-related diseases and extend lifespan. Epigenetics, the study of how environmental factors influence gene expression, sheds more light on the role of genetics in aging.

Customized approaches to anti-aging treatments are made possible by our understanding of the genetic basis of aging. Genetic testing can identify risk factors at an early stage, allowing individuals to take proactive measures like targeted lifestyle modifications, preventive healthcare strategies, and potentially gene-based therapies in the future.

THE IMPACT OF HORMONES ON AGING

Declining hormone levels, including those of progesterone, estrogen, testosterone, and growth hormone, contributes to several aspects of aging. For instance, lower estrogen levels in women during menopause cause bone loss, hot flashes, and an increased risk of cardiovascular disease. Hormones are essential for controlling many physiological processes throughout life, and their levels and balance change with age.

Age-related declines in growth hormone levels impact metabolism, immune system performance, and muscle mass maintenance; in men, testosterone decline is linked to decreased libido, bone density, and muscle mass, as well as increased body fat and cardiovascular risks. Hormonal fluctuations also impact mood, cognitive function, and general vitality in both sexes.

Hormone replacement therapy (HRT), which involves giving hormones to restore levels to those typically seen in younger adults, is a common strategy to lessen the effects of hormonal decline in aging individuals. However, the advantages and risks of HRT vary depending on individual health factors and should be discussed with healthcare providers to determine the most appropriate course of treatment.

The impact of hormones on overall health and quality of life is highlighted by their role in aging. Individuals may be able to reduce age-related symptoms and maximize their well-being as they age by addressing hormonal imbalances through lifestyle modifications or medical interventions such as hormone replacement therapy (HRT).

CHAPTER THREE
BASICS OF SKINCARE
THE VALUE OF A DAILY SKINCARE PROGRAM

A daily skincare routine is essential to having healthy, radiant skin. It helps protect your skin from environmental stressors and cleanses, and hydrates your skin. It also supports your skin's natural renewal process, which promotes a clearer complexion and lowers the risk of breakouts and irritation. By sticking to a daily routine, you create habits that will benefit your skin's long-term health and general well-being.

Cleaning is the first step in any daily skincare routine because it gets rid of all the dirt, oil, and impurities that have accumulated throughout the day or night. It also makes your skin more receptive to the products that come next. After cleansing, toning helps to balance the pH levels of your skin and tightens pores, giving your skin a smoother appearance. Moisturizing is necessary to hydrate your skin and create a barrier against moisture loss, giving your skin a soft and supple texture. Lastly, wearing sunscreen first thing in the morning protects your skin from UV rays that can cause premature aging, sunburns, and skin cancer.

SELECTING PRODUCTS THAT ARE CORRECT FOR YOUR SKIN TYPE

Whether your skin type is oily, dry, sensitive, combination, or prone to acne, selecting skincare products that are appropriate for your skin type will help to address specific concerns and optimize results. For oily skin, look for non-comedogenic, oil-free products that control oil production without clogging pores. For dry skin, look for richer, hydrating formulations that contain ingredients like hyaluronic acid and ceramides to replenish moisture and strengthen the skin barrier.

Patch testing new products before full application is crucial to ensure compatibility and prevent potential allergic reactions or sensitivities. Combination skin requires a balanced approach, using products that hydrate dry areas without aggravating oiliness in others. Sensitive skin needs gentle, fragrance-free products that soothe and minimize irritation, while acne-prone skin benefits from ingredients like salicylic acid or benzoyl peroxide to unclog pores and reduce breakouts.

TIPS FOR CLEANING, SCRUBBING, AND MOISTURIZING

Any skincare routine must begin with cleansing, which removes impurities and prepares the skin for subsequent treatments. Wash your face twice a day, in the morning and at night, using a gentle cleanser appropriate for your skin type.

Exfoliation, performed two to three times a week, helps to remove dead skin cells and reveal smoother, brighter skin. Use a chemical exfoliant, such as glycolic acid, for a gentle yet effective renewal, or use a physical exfoliant with fine particles for a deeper cleanse.

To keep skin hydrated and stop moisture loss throughout the day, moisturize your skin using the type of moisturizer that works best for you (richer for dry skin, lighter for oily skin). After cleansing or exfoliating, apply the moisturizer right away while the skin is still damp to seal in moisture. You should also think about using active ingredients in your moisturizer, such as vitamin C for antioxidant protection or retinoids for anti-aging benefits, applying them first to maximize their effectiveness.

SUNSCREEN USE AND ITS IMPORTANCE

Sunscreen is a must-have for preventing premature aging and lowering the risk of skin cancer. UV rays can pass through windows on cloudy days, so make sure you apply it every day. Look for a broad-spectrum sunscreen with an SPF of 30 or higher, and generously apply it to all exposed areas of your skin, including your hands, neck, and face. Reapply every two hours, or more frequently if you're swimming or perspiring, to ensure maximum protection.

Apart from applying sunscreen, you should also look for shade during the hours of greatest sunlight, which are usually from 10 AM to 4 PM, and wear protective apparel like hats and sunglasses. Sun protection is particularly important if you engage in outdoor activities or spend a lot of time in direct sunlight. Sunscreen is an essential part of any daily skincare routine that helps protect your skin from damage and preserve its youthful appearance.

ESSENTIALS OF A NIGHTTIME SKINCARE ROUTINE

To promote cell turnover and rejuvenation, your skin needs to be replenished and repaired while you sleep. To start, wash your face thoroughly to get rid of all the pollutants, makeup, and sunscreen that have accumulated throughout the day. Use a gentle cleanser that is appropriate for your skin type to prevent stripping natural oils. After cleaning, use a toner to balance the pH levels of your skin and get ready for nighttime treatments.

Moisturizing is essential to lock in hydration and support the skin's natural repair process. Choose a nourishing night cream or moisturizer with ingredients like peptides or hyaluronic acid to hydrate and plump the skin. Nighttime is ideal for applying targeted treatments like serums or retinoids, which penetrate deeply to address specific concerns like fine lines, wrinkles, or hyperpigmentation. These treatments work overnight to promote collagen production and enhance skin renewal.

Use an eye cream for sensitive issues around the eyes, such as puffiness or dark circles. Lastly, use a sleeping mask or overnight treatment to boost hydration and optimize the benefits of your nighttime skincare routine. When you follow a nightly skincare routine, your skin is rejuvenated and you wake up with a complexion that is more radiant and youthful.

CHAPTER FOUR

UNDERSTANDING ANTI-AGING COMPONENTS

SUMMARY OF THE PRINCIPAL ANTI-AGING COMPONENTS

Anyone who wants to improve their skincare routine and effectively fight signs of aging must understand the key anti-aging ingredients. These ingredients are powerful allies in the fight for youthful skin, each with its benefits and applications. Retinoids are well-known for their ability to speed up cell turnover, which smoothes fine lines and wrinkles over time. Vitamins C and E are important for antioxidant defense, protecting skin from damage and encouraging the production of collagen for firmer, more resilient skin. Hyaluronic acid is highly regarded for its ability to hydrate skin cells, plumping them and giving them a dewy glow. Peptides are highly valued for their role in stimulating collagen synthesis and improving skin.

RETINOIDS: THEIR ADVANTAGES

Retinoids are vitamin A derivatives that are well known for their transformative effects on aging skin. They work by accelerating cell turnover, which means they help shed old, damaged skin cells more quickly to reveal newer, smoother skin underneath. Over time, this process improves skin texture and helps to reduce the appearance of fine lines, wrinkles, and age spots. Additionally, retinoids stimulate the production of collagen, a crucial protein that maintains the structure and elasticity of skin, leading to firmer and more youthful-looking skin. Beginners should start with lower concentrations to build tolerance and gradually increase usage to avoid potential irritation. It is best to incorporate retinoids into nighttime skincare routines.

THE VALUE OF VITAMINS E AND C

Together, these vitamins form a strong defense against oxidative stress, enhancing skin's resilience and youthful appearance.

Vitamin C, also known as ascorbic acid, is vital for collagen synthesis, which is necessary for skin elasticity and firmness. It also brightens skin tone by reducing hyperpigmentation and promoting a more even complexion. On the other hand, vitamin E shields the skin from environmental damage caused by free radicals, such as pollution and UV radiation. Its antioxidant action helps prevent premature aging and supports the skin's natural repair processes.

THE FUNCTION OF HYALURONIC ACID IN SKINCARE

A naturally occurring substance in the skin, hyaluronic acid maintains hydration levels by binding water molecules, plumping skin cells, and smoothing fine lines and wrinkles. Its lightweight texture makes it suitable for all skin types, including sensitive and acne-prone skin. Adding hyaluronic acid serums or moisturizers to daily skincare routines can replenish skin's moisture barrier, enhancing suppleness and elasticity. Hyaluronic acid also helps to improve skin texture and radiance, giving skin a youthful, dewy appearance. Regular use of hyaluronic acid-infused products can provide long-lasting hydration benefits.

PEPTIDES AND HOW THEY AFFECT SKIN AGING

Using peptides in skincare routines can help improve skin texture, minimize fine lines, and enhance overall skin resilience. Peptide-infused serums or creams are formulated to penetrate deeply into the skin, delivering potent anti-aging benefits. Over time, peptides can contribute to a more youthful complexion, making them a valuable addition to any anti-aging skincare regimen. Peptides are short chains of amino acids that play a crucial role in collagen synthesis and skin rejuvenation. They act as messengers, signaling skin cells to produce more collagen, which is essential for maintaining skin structure, elasticity, and firmness.

CHAPTER FIVE

GOOD LIVING PRACTICES

DIET IS IMPORTANT FOR PREVENTING AGING

Incorporating foods high in vitamins C and E, such as citrus fruits and avocados, promotes collagen production and skin elasticity. Omega-3 fatty acids, found in fish and flaxseeds, are crucial for maintaining skin hydration and suppleness. Finally, incorporating lean proteins supports skin repair and regeneration processes. All of these factors contribute to the aging process, so it is important to maintain a balanced diet.

A plate full of colorful fruits, vegetables, whole grains, and lean proteins guarantees a steady supply of vital nutrients for vibrant, youthful skin. Reducing sugar intake and processed foods is also important because they can cause glycation, a process where sugars bind to proteins like collagen and cause skin to lose elasticity and firmness.

TOP FOODS FOR RADIANT SKIN

Some foods are especially good for looking younger. Leafy greens like spinach and kale provide vitamins A, C, and E, which are important for collagen production and maintaining skin elasticity. Nuts and seeds like almonds and sunflower seeds offer omega-3 fatty acids and vitamin E, which support skin hydration and protect against sun damage. Berries like blueberries and strawberries are rich in antioxidants that protect skin cells from oxidative stress and premature aging.

Consuming foods high in beta-carotene, such as sweet potatoes and carrots, increases the skin's natural defense against sun damage and encourages a healthy glow. Lean proteins, such as fish, chicken, and legumes, help repair skin tissues and preserve skin structure. Finally, drinking plenty of water and eating foods high in water, such as cucumbers and watermelon, keeps skin hydrated and youthful.

THE VALUE OF HYDRATION

Maintaining proper hydration is essential to having healthy, youthful-looking skin. Water helps the body eliminate toxins, prevents dehydration, and promotes a clear complexion. Sufficient hydration improves skin elasticity, which minimizes the appearance of fine lines and wrinkles. It also facilitates the delivery of vital nutrients to skin cells, which contributes to a youthful, radiant appearance.

In addition to drinking water, eating fruits and vegetables that are high in water content raises your body's level of hydration. Cucumbers, tomatoes, and oranges are just a few examples of foods high in water content that keep skin hydrated and supple. Herbal teas and coconut water are good sources of extra nutrients that promote skin health.

EXERCISE'S ANTI-AGING PROPERTIES

Frequent exercise is an effective anti-aging strategy that benefits the body as well as the skin. Aerobic exercises, such as cycling or jogging, improve skin tone and texture by reducing inflammation and encouraging sweat-induced detoxification. Physical activity also increases blood circulation, which delivers oxygen and essential nutrients to skin cells, which promotes collagen production and enhances skin elasticity.

A regular exercise regimen not only improves overall health but also makes you look younger and more vibrant. Strength training exercises, like weightlifting or yoga, help maintain muscle mass and prevent sagging skin as you age. Exercise also reduces stress levels, which can contribute to premature aging signs like wrinkles and dull complexion.

SLEEP IS CRUCIAL FOR MAINTAINING SKIN HEALTH

Appropriate sleep duration enables the skin to recuperate from daily environmental stressors like UV radiation and pollution. Sleep deprivation can raise cortisol levels, which accelerate the breakdown of collagen and contribute to the appearance of wrinkles and fine lines. Quality sleep is essential for skin repair, rejuvenation, and general health.

A regular sleep schedule and good sleep hygiene, like establishing a relaxing bedtime routine and providing a comfortable sleep environment, support optimal skin health. Adequate rest enhances skin's natural glow and resilience, contributing to a youthful appearance over time. Furthermore, sleep deprivation affects skin hydration levels, making the skin appear dull, dry, and less resilient.

CHAPTER SIX

NON-SURGICAL AGE-REDUCTION METHODS

SYNOPSIS OF NON-INVASIVE THERAPIES

A variety of less invasive procedures, such as chemical peels, microdermabrasion, laser treatments, facial massages, microcurrent therapy, and LED therapy, are commonly used as non-surgical anti-aging treatments. These procedures are intended to improve skin texture, tone, and overall appearance through an approach that is less aggressive and requires less downtime.

Both chemical peels and microdermabrasion can improve skin radiance and smoothness without requiring surgery. Chemical peels involve applying a chemical solution to the skin, which exfoliates the outer layer and stimulates cell turnover. This process helps to improve skin clarity, reduce fine lines, and even out skin tone. Microdermabrasion uses fine crystals or a diamond-tipped wand to gently exfoliate the skin, removing dead skin cells and stimulating collagen production.

Targeting specific skin concerns like wrinkles, age spots, and uneven pigmentation, laser treatments use focused light energy to stimulate collagen production and promote skin renewal. Customized to each patient's skin type and concerns, laser therapies deliver precise and effective results. Usually requiring multiple sessions to achieve the best results, laser treatments are a flexible choice for those looking to gradually improve the appearance of their skin.

BENEFITS OF MICRODERMABRASION AND CHEMICAL PEELS

Beginners interested in non-invasive anti-aging treatments can benefit from chemical peels and microdermabrasion in several ways. Chemical peels effectively treat skin issues like wrinkles, fine lines, acne scars, and uneven pigmentation by removing damaged outer layers of skin, which encourages the growth of new, smoother skin and improves overall skin tone and texture. Chemical peels come in a variety of forms, from superficial to deep, allowing for treatment customization based on individual skin concerns and sensitivity levels.

In contrast, microdermabrasion uses fine crystals or a diamond-tipped wand to gently exfoliate the skin's surface. This mechanical exfoliation promotes collagen production and circulation, which improves skin elasticity and gives the appearance of younger skin. Microdermabrasion is appropriate for mild to moderate skin imperfections and is frequently suggested as a maintenance treatment to keep skin looking young and vibrant.

Beginning users can anticipate smoother, brighter skin following treatment, as well as improved absorption of skincare products for increased effectiveness. Both treatments are safe for most skin types and reasonably quick, usually taking less than an hour per session with little discomfort and downtime.

COMPREHENDING LASER PROCEDURES

By stimulating the skin's natural healing process, concentrated light beams are used in advanced non-surgical procedures called laser treatments to target specific skin concerns and promote collagen production.

The deep penetration of laser energy into the skin without damaging the outer layer allows for precise treatment of targeted areas, and the treatments are highly effective in reducing wrinkles, fine lines, sun damage, and age spots.

Abrasive lasers remove thin layers of skin to improve texture and reduce wrinkles; non-ablative lasers heat the underlying layers of skin to stimulate collagen production without causing damage to the surface; fractional lasers cause tiny wounds in the skin to stimulate the body's natural healing response and to promote the formation of new collagen. These are just a few of the different types of laser treatments that are available.

While laser treatments are generally safe and well-tolerated, beginners need to consult with a qualified dermatologist or skincare specialist to determine the most suitable laser treatment based on their skin type and concerns. Typically, multiple sessions spaced several weeks apart are required to achieve optimal results. The number of sessions depends on the severity of the skin condition being treated and the desired outcome.

THE VALUE OF MASSAGES FOR THE FACE

Including gentle manipulation of facial muscles and tissues to improve circulation, encourage lymphatic drainage, and relieve facial tension, facial massages are an essential component of non-invasive anti-aging treatments. By increasing blood flow to the skin, they help deliver oxygen and nutrients to cells, resulting in a healthier and more radiant complexion.

Frequent facial massages are a great complement to any skincare routine because they can reduce puffiness, diminish fine lines, enhance the absorption of skincare products, and stimulate the production of collagen, which over time leads to firmer and more elastic skin. To get the most out of facial massages and achieve comprehensive skin rejuvenation, they are frequently combined with other treatments like moisturizing masks or serums.

Facial massages also help to relieve tension in the facial muscles and promote a feeling of well-being, which can improve the overall health of the skin. They also help to rejuvenate the complexion and give a youthful appearance. Those who are new to massage therapy can learn basic techniques from skincare professionals or incorporate light massage movements into their daily skincare routine for noticeable improvements in skin tone and texture.

ADVANTAGES OF LED THERAPY WITH MICROCURRENT

Microcurrent therapy uses low-level electrical currents to stimulate facial muscles and tissues, resulting in improved muscle tone and firmer skin.

These gentle electrical impulses mimic the body's natural electrical signals, promoting cellular rejuvenation and collagen production. Together, microcurrent and LED therapy are innovative non-invasive treatments that offer unique benefits for enhancing skin elasticity, reducing wrinkles, and improving overall skin tone.

Red and infrared light wavelengths stimulate collagen production and accelerate skin healing, while blue light wavelengths help reduce acne-causing bacteria and improve skin clarity. LED therapy is non-thermal and non-invasive, making it suitable for sensitive skin types and those seeking gentle yet effective skincare treatments. LED therapy uses specific wavelengths of light to penetrate the skin at varying depths, targeting different skin concerns such as acne, inflammation, and signs of aging.

Incorporating microcurrent or LED therapy into a regular skincare routine can help maintain long-term skin health and vitality, making them valuable tools in anti-aging skincare regimens.

Both microcurrent and LED therapies are painless and require no downtime, making them convenient options for beginners looking to improve the appearance of their skin without undergoing surgery. These treatments can be performed in a series of sessions to achieve cumulative benefits, such as enhanced skin firmness, reduced fine lines, and a more youthful complexion.

CHAPTER SEVEN

SURGICAL METHODS FOR ANTI-AGING

WHEN TO THINK ABOUT GETTING SURGERY

It is important to speak with a qualified cosmetic surgeon who can evaluate your suitability for surgery based on your medical history, skin condition, and aesthetic goals. Surgical procedures are often chosen when non-invasive treatments no longer provide the desired results, such as addressing deep wrinkles, sagging skin, or significant facial volume loss that cannot be effectively treated with less invasive methods. Choosing to undergo surgical anti-aging treatments is a significant decision that should be carefully considered. The ideal candidates are typically people who have realistic expectations about the outcomes and are in good overall health.

Surgical anti-aging options can yield more dramatic and long-lasting results than non-surgical treatments, but they also come with recovery time and potential risks like infection, scarring, or complications related to anesthesia. Before committing to surgery, it's important to understand the risks and benefits associated with each procedure. The decision to undergo surgery should be well-informed and based on a thorough discussion with your surgeon about expectations, recovery process, and post-operative care requirements.

SUMMARY OF FACELIFT PROCEDURES AND THEIR VARIATIONS

Facelift surgery, also referred to as rhytidectomy, is a surgical procedure intended to rejuvenate the face by treating deep creases, sagging skin, and loss of muscle tone. There are several facelift techniques, each customized to address specific areas of concern and produce results that look natural. Traditional facelifts involve incisions made around the ears and occasionally along the hairline, allowing the surgeon to remove excess skin, lift and reposition underlying tissues, and smooth out wrinkles.

Mini facelifts are less invasive alternatives that target particular face regions with smaller incisions and shorter recovery periods, making them suitable for patients with mild to moderate signs of aging.

Advanced facelift techniques, like deep plane or SMAS facelifts, aim to lift deeper layers of facial tissues for more thorough rejuvenation. To restore volume and improve facial contours, these procedures are frequently combined with fat grafting or facial implants. Recovery from a facelift usually involves temporary swelling, bruising, and discomfort, which can be controlled with medication and appropriate post-operative care. Over a few weeks, as swelling reduces, results become more refreshed and youthful-looking.

COMPREHENDING FILLERS AND BOTOX

Injecting small amounts of botulinum toxin into specific facial muscles temporarily relaxes the muscles that cause wrinkles and lines, especially those on the forehead, around the eyes (crow's feet), and between the eyebrows (glabellar lines). This prevents wrinkles from deepening over time and smoothes out wrinkles; results usually last three to six months, after which additional treatments may be required to maintain effects. Dermal fillers are another popular non-surgical option for reducing wrinkles, enhancing facial contours, and restoring youthful volume.

Hyaluronic acid-based dermal fillers (e.g., Juvederm, Restylane) are used to plump up lips, smooth out nasolabial folds (smile lines), enhance cheekbones, and improve under-eye hollows. Dermal fillers are injected into specific areas to create a natural-looking fullness and lift. The procedure involves injecting filler into these areas; results are immediate and can last anywhere from six months to two years, depending on the type of filler used and individual metabolism. Like Botox, maintenance treatments are required to maintain results over time.

BENEFITS OF EYELID SURGERY

Lower eyelid surgery focuses on reducing fat deposits and tightening lax skin to eliminate under-eye bags and improve overall eye contour. Eyelid surgery, also known as blepharoplasty, is a surgical procedure intended to rejuvenate the appearance of the eyes by addressing puffiness, drooping eyelids, and under-eye bags. The procedure can also correct ptosis, or drooping eyelids, which may impair vision or create a tired appearance.

Eyelid surgery is thought to be a long-lasting solution for rejuvenating the eyes, with results that can last for many years. Benefits of eyelid surgery include a more alert and youthful appearance, enhanced peripheral vision, and improved self-confidence.

Recovery from eyelid surgery typically involves temporary swelling, bruising, and mild discomfort, which can be managed with cold compresses and prescribed medications. Most patients return to normal activities within one to two weeks, with the final results becoming apparent as the swelling resolves.

LIPOSUCTION FOR SCULPTING THE FACE

A thin tube called a cannula is inserted through small incisions to suction out fat cells, sculpting the desired contours. Liposuction is a surgical procedure that can be used for facial contouring by removing excess fat deposits from areas such as the chin, neck, and jowls. Facial liposuction is ideal for people who have stubborn fat pockets that are resistant to diet and exercise, leading to a more defined jawline and improved facial proportions.

Compression garments may be worn to minimize swelling and support the newly contoured areas. Full results become evident as swelling subsides, revealing a more sculpted and balanced facial appearance. Liposuction can provide long-lasting results with proper diet and exercise maintenance. Common areas treated with facial liposuction include the double chin (submental liposuction) and jowls, creating a slimmer and more defined facial profile. Following surgery, results are visible right away.

Whether restoring facial volume, lifting sagging tissues, or refining facial contours, these surgical anti-aging options offer effective solutions for people looking to rejuvenate their appearance and address specific aging concerns. Each procedure is customized to meet different aesthetic goals; speaking with a board-certified cosmetic surgeon is crucial to determining the most appropriate treatment plan based on individual needs, ensuring safe and satisfactory outcomes.

CHAPTER EIGHT

MALE ANTI-AGING

DISTINCTIVE OBSTACLES IN THE FIELD OF ANTI-AGING FOR MEN

Men's skin structure, hormonal fluctuations, and lifestyle choices all present distinct obstacles when it comes to anti-aging. Among these is the thicker, oilier skin type of men, which can cause problems such as acne, enlarged pores, and more noticeable wrinkles and lines. Additionally, men's levels of collagen and elastin, which support the skin structurally but diminish with age, are also generally higher in men.

Understanding these subtleties can help men adopt effective anti-aging tactics tailored to their needs, assuring better outcomes and improved skin health over time.

MEN'S SKINCARE ROUTINES

To combat signs of aging, men's skin needs a comprehensive skincare routine that begins with cleansing with products made to remove excess oil and impurities without drying out the skin. Exfoliation follows cleansing to help slough off dead skin cells and promote cell turnover, revealing smoother, more youthful-looking skin. Gentle yet effective exfoliants that contain alpha hydroxy acids (AHAs) or beta hydroxy acids (BHAs) are recommended for men.

After exfoliation, hydration is essential. Restoring moisture to the skin, improving its texture, and minimizing the appearance of fine lines and wrinkles can be achieved by using a moisturizer enhanced with antioxidants and anti-aging ingredients such as retinol.

DIETARY CONSIDERATIONS FOR MALE SKIN HEALTH

A well-balanced diet is essential for maintaining male skin health and preventing internal aging signs. Antioxidant-rich foods like berries, leafy greens, and nuts help prevent oxidative stress, which speeds up aging and neutralizes free radicals. Omega-3 fatty acids, which are found in fatty fish like salmon and walnut nuts, help hydrate and elasticity of the skin, which minimizes the appearance of wrinkles.

In addition, drinking lots of water throughout the day helps to maintain moisture levels and flush out toxins, which in turn helps to promote healthy skin. Limiting intake of processed foods, sugars, and alcohol can also help to improve skin health because these substances can exacerbate inflammation and speed up the aging process.

Regular exercise increases blood circulation, delivering vital nutrients and oxygen to skin cells, promoting a healthy complexion and youthful glow. It also helps to reduce stress levels, which can contribute to premature aging by inducing inflammatory responses in the body. Men's overall health and appearance can be enhanced by incorporating strength training exercises, like weightlifting, to maintain muscle mass and tone.

MALE-SPECIFIC TREATMENTS AND PROCEDURES

Apart from skincare regimens and lifestyle modifications, there are specific treatments and procedures designed to address age-related concerns in men. A popular choice is laser therapy, which targets wrinkles, age spots, and uneven skin tone by promoting skin renewal and stimulating collagen production. Microdermabrasion is another efficacious treatment that exfoliates the skin and minimizes the appearance of fine lines and age spots.

Understanding these options enables men to make educated decisions about their anti-aging journey, achieving desired results with confidence and efficacy. For more advanced signs of aging, cosmetic procedures like botox injections or dermal fillers can smooth out wrinkles and restore facial volume. These treatments are administered by qualified professionals and tailored to meet individual aesthetic goals.

CHAPTER NINE

ANTI-AGING FOR VARIOUS TYPES OF SKIN

RECOGNIZING AGING ISSUES FOR VARIOUS SKIN TYPES

Depending on the type of skin—dry, oily, sensitive, or combination—aging affects it differently. Dry skin is prone to fine lines and early loss of elasticity because it retains less moisture.

Oily skin, which produces too much sebum, may face wrinkles later but is more likely to have enlarged pores and uneven texture. Sensitive skin is more likely to experience redness, irritation, and premature aging as a result of outside factors like harsh products or weather changes.

For optimal results, each skin type needs to be treated differently to address specific concerns related to aging. For example, oily skin needs lightweight, non-comedogenic products that control oil production while preventing clogged pores and breakouts;

sensitive skin needs gentle, fragrance-free formulations that soothe irritation and fortify the skin barrier against premature aging; and combination skin benefits from a balanced approach that uses targeted treatments for each area to maintain overall skin health and prevent uneven aging signs.

Knowing how various skin types are affected by aging enables people to select skincare products and regimens that suit their individual needs. By recognizing particular issues early on and implementing targeted anti-aging techniques, people can eventually attain healthier, more youthful-looking skin. Including these understandings into regular skincare routines guarantees that signs of aging are reduced and skin, no matter what type, remains resilient and radiant.

CUSTOMIZING SKINCARE PROGRAMS FOR SENSITIVE, OILY, AND DRY SKIN:

The first step in developing a successful skincare routine is identifying and meeting the specific needs of oily, dry, and sensitive skin types. Oily skin needs lightweight moisturizers and cleansers without alcohol, which balance sebum production without clogging pores. Adding exfoliants to the mix helps to refine skin texture and prevent acne breakouts. Sensitive skin needs hypoallergenic and fragrance-free products that reduce redness and soothe irritation. Staying away from harsh ingredients like alcohol and sulfates is essential to prevent exacerbating sensitivity.

Customizing skincare routines to suit individual skin types allows people to effectively manage issues like dryness, excess oil, and sensitivity while promoting overall skin health and resilience. Individuals with dry skin benefit from hydrating cleansers, rich moisturizers, and weekly exfoliation to remove dead skin cells gently.

Oily skin needs oil-controlling cleansers, lightweight moisturizers, and regular exfoliation to prevent buildup and congestion. Sensitive skin thrives with gentle cleansers, calming moisturizers, and minimalistic routines that minimize irritation.

Skin type-specific skincare regimen adjustments yield the best results when it comes to addressing aging issues and preserving the health of the skin. By choosing products and techniques that are appropriate for their needs, people can maximize the effectiveness of their anti-aging regimen and attain smoother, more youthful-looking skin.

Including these customized approaches into daily skin care routines promotes long-term skin resilience and vitality, enabling people to face aging with confidence and effectiveness.

ANTI-AGING ADVICE FOR SKIN TYPE: COMBINATION

Combination skin poses particular difficulties in controlling signs of aging in distinct facial zones. The T-zone (forehead, nose, and chin) is typically oily, whereas the cheeks and other areas may be dry or normal.

Customizing anti-aging strategies requires striking a balance between hydration and sebum control to effectively address varying needs. Lightweight, non-comedogenic moisturizers help maintain moisture balance without aggravating oiliness in the T-zone. Targeted treatments, such as serums containing antioxidants or retinoids, can target specific aging concerns in distinct facial areas, thereby promoting overall resilience and homogeneity of skin.

Combination skin needs a balanced approach to address specific needs in both oily and dry areas. Gentle cleansers, hydrating toners, and targeted treatments are part of a routine that ensures comprehensive care without disrupting the balance of the skin.

Weekly exfoliation improves the texture and clarity of the skin on all facial zones by removing dead skin cells and encouraging cell turnover. By incorporating these customized strategies into their daily skincare routines, people with combination skin can effectively manage signs of aging while promoting overall skin health and vitality.

Accepting these anti-aging tips empowers people to achieve smoother, more youthful-looking skin while adapting to the changing needs of combination skin over time. Understanding the unique characteristics of combination skin is necessary to navigate its complexities and address aging concerns with targeted solutions.

People can maintain skin health and resilience across all facial zones by incorporating customized skincare routines and products that balance hydration and oil control.

THE VALUE OF PH EQUILIBRIUM IN SKINCARE

The natural pH of the skin functions as a barrier against harmful bacteria and environmental stressors; using skincare products with a pH similar to the skin's acidity helps maintain this barrier function, preventing moisture loss and maintaining optimal skin health. Deviations in pH can disrupt the skin's acid mantle, leading to dryness, sensitivity, and accelerated aging signs like fine lines and wrinkles. Therefore, the pH level of skincare products and formulations is important for maintaining skin health and preventing premature aging.

Achieving effective skincare results and optimizing product efficacy requires product selection that respects the skin's natural pH balance. pH-balanced cleansers preserve the skin's moisture barrier and minimize irritation by gently removing impurities; pH-balanced toners help the skin return to its natural acidity after cleansing, making it more receptive to subsequent skincare products; and incorporating pH-balanced moisturizers and serums into daily routines promotes overall skin health by hydrating the skin and preventing premature aging signs linked to pH imbalance.

Keeping the pH balance of skincare routines optimal supports healthy skin function and effectively supports anti-aging efforts.

People can improve their skin's ability to retain moisture, fend off outside stressors, and look younger by choosing pH-balanced products customized to their specific skin needs.

Including pH-conscious skincare practices into daily routines guarantees that the skin stays resilient, balanced, and ready to fight signs of aging over time.

SELECTING ITEMS DEPENDING ON SKIN TYPE

Achieving effective anti-aging results requires choosing skincare products that are specific to each skin type. For example, dry skin needs rich, hydrating formulations that replenish moisture and restore elasticity; look for ingredients like hyaluronic acid and shea butter, which deeply hydrate and nourish dry skin without leaving a greasy residue.

On the other hand, oily skin needs lightweight, oil-free products that minimize pores and control shine; salicylic acid and niacinamide help regulate sebum production and prevent breakouts, promoting a matte finish.

Gentle, fragrance-free formulas that reduce irritation and fortify the skin barrier are ideal for sensitive skin. Look for products that are labeled hypoallergenic and non-comedogenic to reduce the likelihood of allergic reactions and breakouts.

Products that are versatile and address both oily and dry areas without upsetting the balance are best for combination skin. Look for moisturizers and serums that are made to hydrate dry patches and mattify oily zones, providing all-over facial care.

People can effectively optimize their anti-aging regimen and attain their desired results by selecting skincare products that are tailored to their skin types. These customized product choices guarantee that every skin type receives targeted care to address specific concerns like dryness, oiliness, sensitivity, and combination needs.

Including these customized approaches into daily skin care routines supports long-term skin health and resilience, enabling people to face aging with confidence and achieve smoother, more youthful-looking skin over time.

CHAPTER TEN
FAQS & FREQUENTLY ASKED QUESTIONS

HANDLING FINE LINES AND WRINKLES

Naturally occurring wrinkles and fine lines can be effectively managed with the right skincare and treatments. One of the most important strategies is to follow a daily skincare routine that includes moisturizing and using products containing antioxidants, retinoids, and peptides. These ingredients help stimulate collagen production, which is crucial for maintaining skin elasticity and reducing the appearance of wrinkles. You should also use sunscreen every day because UV rays accelerate the aging process of the skin.

Injectable treatments like Botox and dermal fillers, which help relax muscles and fill in wrinkles, respectively, are another effective way to treat specific areas of the skin. For example, microdermabrasion and chemical peels can help exfoliate the skin and improve its texture by removing dead skin cells and promoting cell turnover, resulting in smoother and more youthful-looking skin.

In addition to these treatments, healthy lifestyle choices like eating a diet high in antioxidants and drinking plenty of water are essential. Refraining from smoking and excessive sun exposure also helps to prevent wrinkles from getting worse and preserve the quality of your skin overall.

HOW TO HANDLE HYPERPIGMENTATION AND AGE SPOTS

Age spots and hyperpigmentation are prevalent issues that can be effectively managed with a variety of treatment approaches. One such approach is the use of skincare products that contain ingredients such as hydroquinone, kojic acid, vitamin C, and niacinamide. These ingredients function by preventing the production of melanin and gradually promoting even skin tone.

Targeting resistant age spots and hyperpigmentation can also be effectively achieved with in-office procedures like chemical peels and laser therapy, which use concentrated light to break down pigmented cells and reveal clearer skin. Chemical peels involve applying a chemical solution to exfoliate the skin.

Keeping up a regular skincare regimen is essential to preventing the formation of new age spots. Applying broad-spectrum sunscreen every day protects the skin from UV rays, which can aggravate pigmentation problems.

HANDLING DROOPING SKIN

Although it is a normal aspect of aging, sagging skin can be controlled with a variety of non-surgical and surgical treatments. Non-surgical options include skincare products that contain peptides and hyaluronic acid, which help to improve the elasticity and hydration of the skin by gradually increasing the production of collagen and firmness in the skin.

Radiofrequency therapy and ultrasound skin tightening are two effective procedures for more advanced sagging. They work by heating the skin's deeper layers with energy, which stimulates the production of collagen and tightens loose skin without the need for surgery. Another option is thread lifting, which involves inserting biodegradable threads beneath the skin to lift and support sagging areas.

When surgical intervention is warranted, procedures such as neck lifts and facelifts can yield remarkable outcomes by tightening underlying tissues and removing excess skin. It is imperative to consult with a board-certified plastic surgeon or dermatologist to determine the best course of action based on specific goals and skin conditions.

HANDLING PUFFINESS AND UNDER-EYE BAGS

Using cool compresses or chilled tea bags to reduce swelling and constrict blood vessels is an effective home remedy for under-eye bags and puffiness caused by aging, allergies, genetics, and fluid retention. Additionally, applying eye creams containing antioxidants, peptides, and caffeine can help improve circulation and reduce fluid buildup.

Dermal fillers and platelet-rich plasma (PRP) injections are two treatments that can yield noticeable results for more persistent under-eye bags. Dermal fillers plump up hollow areas under the eyes, while PRP injections use the patient's blood plasma to stimulate collagen production and rejuvenate the under-eye area.

Procedures such as fractional CO_2 laser treatments and laser resurfacing can help tighten and smooth the skin if skin laxity is a contributing factor to under-eye bags.

HOW TO AVOID AND HANDLE DARK CIRCLES

Genetics sleep deprivation, allergies, and thinning skin can all contribute to dark circles under the eyes.

Managing allergies, adhering to a regular sleep schedule, and using eye creams with ingredients like vitamin C, vitamin K, and peptides can all help minimize the appearance of under-eye discoloration and improve the texture of the skin.

Chemical peels and microneedling, two in-office procedures that help lighten pigmentation and improve overall skin tone, can also help reduce dark circles. Chemical peels exfoliate the skin and encourage cell turnover, while microneedling stimulates collagen production and improves the absorption of topical treatments.

Intense pulsed light (IPL) and laser therapy are two efficient ways to target stubborn pigmentation under the eyes for more focused outcomes. They produce skin that is brighter and more even-toned by breaking down melanin and promoting the creation of collagen.

CHAPTER ELEVEN

ANTI-AGING TRENDS FOR THE FUTURE

TECHNOLOGICAL ADVANCEMENTS IN SKINCARE

The way we approach anti-aging treatments is being revolutionized by advances in skincare technology, which offer sophisticated solutions that address a variety of skin types and concerns. One of the biggest developments in this regard is the combination of artificial intelligence (AI) and machine learning in skincare diagnostics; AI-powered tools are capable of accurately diagnosing skin conditions and recommending customized treatments based on individual needs. For example, dermatological apps that are AI-enabled can evaluate wrinkles, fine lines, and skin elasticity and direct users toward appropriate anti-aging procedures or products.

The use of nanotechnology in skincare formulations is another noteworthy advancement. Nanoparticles allow active ingredients to penetrate the skin more deeply, increasing their effectiveness in targeting signs of aging such as hyperpigmentation or loss of firmness. This technology guarantees minimal side effects and enhances the delivery of antioxidants and peptides, making it appropriate for sensitive skin types. Additionally, wearable skincare devices with sensors can monitor environmental factors and skin hydration levels, providing real-time data for customized skincare routines.

Developments in light-based therapies, like laser and LED light therapy, have also gained popularity in anti-aging skincare. While fractional laser treatments target specific skin layers to improve texture and tone, effectively addressing issues like age spots and acne scars, LED light therapy stimulates collagen production and reduces inflammation, promoting smoother and more youthful-looking skin. These non-invasive technologies are still evolving, providing safer and more accessible alternatives to traditional surgical procedures for anti-aging.

NEW DEVELOPMENTS IN ANTI-AGING THERAPIES

A trend worth noting is the rise of regenerative medicine in skin care, which uses stem cells and growth factors to rejuvenate aging skin. Stem cell therapy promotes tissue regeneration and repair, enhancing skin elasticity and reducing wrinkles over time. This approach is gaining traction because it can harness the body's natural healing processes without invasive surgery. Emerging trends in anti-aging treatments reflect a shift towards holistic approaches that combine medical expertise with natural and minimally invasive techniques.

The use of cosmeceuticals and nutraceuticals in anti-aging skincare is another noteworthy trend. These formulations combine pharmaceutical-grade ingredients with nutritional supplements, providing powerful antioxidants and vitamins necessary for skin health. Nutraceuticals, such as hyaluronic acid and collagen peptide supplements, support skin hydration and elasticity from the inside out and enhance topical skincare regimens. Cosmeceuticals, on the other hand, use active ingredients like retinoids and peptides to effectively target particular signs of aging.

Combination therapies, which combine various anti-aging modalities for optimal results, have also gained popularity in recent years. For example, microneedling combined with PRP (Platelet-Rich Plasma) therapy improves texture and firmness by leveraging the skin's natural healing response. Similarly, injectable treatments, like Botox and dermal fillers, are being customized to achieve natural-looking results while addressing individual aesthetic goals. These trends emphasize customized approaches catered to each patient's unique skincare needs and aging concerns.

THE VALUE OF CUSTOMIZED SKINCARE

Since each person's skin is different and needs a customized solution for best results, personalized skincare has gained importance in anti-aging treatments.

The first step in a customized skincare routine is a thorough skin assessment performed by a skincare professional or dermatologist. The assessment usually entails analyzing skin type, identifying specific concerns like wrinkles or sagging, and evaluating environmental factors that may impact skin health.

Personalized skincare has advanced with the introduction of genetic testing, which enables practitioners to know a patient's genetic predispositions to aging and tailor treatments accordingly. For example, genetic analysis can identify variations in antioxidant defense mechanisms or collagen production, which can inform the choice of specific skincare procedures or products. Additionally, technological advancements like 3D skin imaging allow for precise treatment planning by providing detailed visual assessments of skin texture and hydration levels.

Beyond product recommendations, personalized skincare also involves lifestyle modifications that support skin health. Dietary changes to improve skin hydration and elasticity, as well as lifestyle adjustments to lessen environmental stressors like pollution or UV exposure, are examples of lifestyle modifications that are part of personalized skincare. Integrative approaches, which combine professional treatments with at-home skincare regimens, enable people to proactively manage aging concerns while preserving overall skin health and resilience.

ECO-FRIENDLY METHODS FOR DELAYING AGING

A major component of sustainability is the use of eco-friendly packaging materials and reducing carbon footprints during product manufacturing and distribution. Brands are increasingly choosing recyclable or biodegradable packaging options to minimize waste and support environmentally responsible practices. Sustainable practices in anti-aging focus on minimizing environmental impact while promoting ethical sourcing and production methods across the skincare industry.

In addition, natural and organic components from wild harvesting or sustainable agriculture are given priority in sustainable skincare formulations. Plant-based actives and botanical extracts provide potent anti-aging benefits while reducing chemical exposure and environmental damage. Sustainable sourcing guarantees biodiversity and ecosystem preservation, so skincare decisions are in line with international conservation initiatives.

Sustainable anti-aging practices extend beyond product formulation and include ethical aspects like transparent supply chains and fair trade partnerships with local communities. Fostering fair labor practices and empowering communities involved in ingredient sourcing are two ways that the skincare industry is socially responsible. By advancing sustainability, skincare brands fulfill consumer demand for environmentally friendly products while also upholding moral standards that benefit people and the environment.

INTERNATIONAL VIEWS ON RESEARCH ON ANTI-AGING

International collaborations foster knowledge exchange and scientific advancements that benefit the world's aging population. Research institutions worldwide are conducting studies on cutting-edge anti-aging technologies, ranging from biotechnology and regenerative medicine to cultural practices that promote longevity and vitality. Global perspectives on anti-aging research highlight collaborative efforts and diverse approaches to addressing aging concerns across different regions and cultures.

Asian skincare traditions, for instance, emphasize herbal ingredients like ginseng and green tea known for their antioxidant properties and skin-rejuvenating effects. These cultural insights inspire the development of hybrid skincare formulations that blend ancient wisdom with modern scientific research, catering to diverse consumer needs globally. Cultural perspectives on aging influence skincare practices and preferences, with traditional remedies and rituals playing a significant role in anti-aging regimens.

Global perspectives enable anti-aging research to advance holistic approaches to healthy aging globally. Additionally, global anti-aging research initiatives prioritize inclusivity and diversity in clinical trials to guarantee treatments are effective across different skin tones and ethnicities. This approach not only improves treatment outcomes but also promotes equity in access to cutting-edge skincare solutions.

www.ingramcontent.com/pod-product-compliance
Lightning Source LLC
Chambersburg PA
CBHW061254250726
48653CB00002B/651